a morning cup of
stretching ™

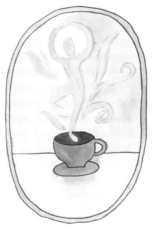

This edition published for Sweetwater Press by arrangement with
Crane Hill Publishers.

ISBN 1-58173-261-9

Book design by Miles Parsons
Illustrations by Tim Rocks
Cover art by Tim Rocks and Ernie Eldredge

Printed in Italy

10   9   8   7   6   5   4   3   2   1

a morning cup of
stretching™

one 15-minute routine to wake up
your mind and body

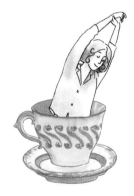

Beth Pierpoint, M.S.P.T.

SWEET
WATER
PRESS

Acknowledgments

I am grateful for the wonderful people I have met in my career. I have been fortunate to work with international dignitaries, world-class physicians, and national sports figures, and I have been blessed to learn from all of them.

My patients have taught me the best lessons in life. So this book is dedicated to them. My career would not be nearly so fulfilling had they not touched my life.

I want to thank my father, for instilling in me the belief that I could do anything.

I also want to thank God and my family and friends, who have supported me throughout my career as well as during the writing of this book. Without them, none of this would have been possible.

Contents

The Case for Stretching

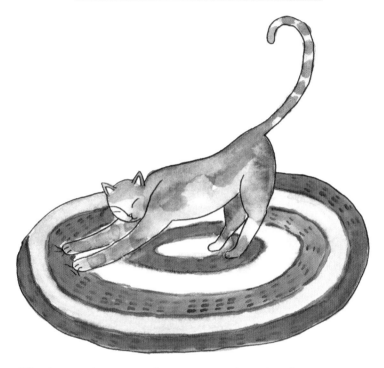

Watch your dog or cat the next time she wakes from a nap. The first thing she'll do is take a good long stretch. Nothing feels better than a full-body stretch after awakening. We humans do it, too (although not nearly often enough). This book takes that great feeling and builds on it for each muscle group.

It's easy to make a case for daily stretching. People who build stretching into their daily routines maintain strength and flexibility, have better posture, and experience far fewer aches and pains and other degenerative problems as they age. Those who take the time to stretch at work have fewer headaches, and reduce the risk of carpal tunnel syndrome, low back pain, and other problems that result from repetitive-motion type jobs.

Stretching became popular during the aerobics craze of the 1980s, when fitness instructors began recommending stretching at the beginning of exercise programs. But physical therapists have long known that a simple stretching routine all by itself is extremely beneficial.

I designed the routine in this book for men and women of all ages. The combination of stretches can be performed in about 15 minutes. The book contains ideas for stretches you can do first thing in the morning, or anytime during the day – at home, or on the job.

We can't truly address stretching and its benefits without considering posture. And posture is almost always directly linked to workspace, where most of us spend the bulk of the day. Later in the book, I offer suggestions and inexpensive solutions for making sure your workstation fits you. Too often, people mold to fit their workstations, when it should be the other way around. That leads to bad posture at work, which means eight to ten hours of damage done, day in and day out.

A little preventive medicine can go a long way toward correcting this problem. That's what I hope this book will do for you – help keep your muscles strong and flexible, while helping you prevent muscular aches and pains. I think you'll be pleasantly surprised at what *A Morning Cup of Stretching* can do.

Beth Pierpoint

Stretching — It's a Natural!

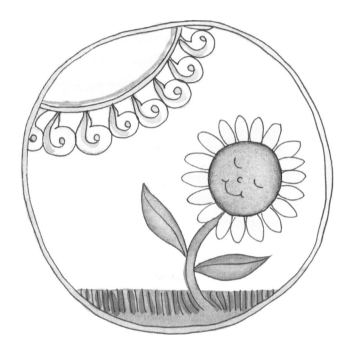

I'm sold on stretching. It's good for you. It comes naturally to us all. It helps you feel better, regardless of whether you do it on its own or as a lead-in to another exercise regimen.

I've witnessed the benefits of stretching throughout my career as a physical therapist. Typically my patients have injuries that result from either neurological damage or muscular and skeletal injury. I've used stretching for years as an essential baseline component of all their rehabilitation programs, including those of injured professional athletes in the LPGA and World Wrestling Federation, as well as players from NBA, NFL, and other pro teams including the Atlanta

Braves, St. Louis Cardinals, Boston Red Sox, Tampa Bay Devil Rays, Chicago White Sox, Chicago Bulls, Indiana Pacers, and the Washington Redskins.

My love of sports and fitness began when I was growing up in Reno, Nevada. I really enjoyed competing, and at nine years old, I started playing golf and softball. In 1983, I was offered a softball scholarship to the University of Nevada-Reno.

I developed an interest in physical therapy while taking sports medicine classes at the University of Nevada. To gain the experience I'd need to qualify for physical therapy school, I worked at several physical therapy practices that offered pain management and sports medicine, and I supervised patients undergoing exercise programs. I also taught aerobics and other exercises at the YWCA in Reno.

I graduated from physical therapy school in Forest Grove, Oregon, in 1994, and began my professional career. Rather than settling down in one city, I decided to tour the United States as a consulting physical therapist. So I packed my bags and took off in my Honda CRX two-seater. For about a year and a half, I filled in with 13-week stints at various health care facilities.

When I found a job at a prominent rehabilitation and sports medicine hospital in Birmingham, Alabama, I decided it was time to quit the road. I particularly enjoyed my work in Birmingham because it allowed me to treat patients with all types of needs and challenges, including those resulting from orthopedic injuries, arthritis, multiple sclerosis, strokes, and spinal cord injuries.

As I mentioned earlier, stretching has always been a part of my physical therapy treatment regimes for patients. However, as I have grown older and noticed a "sag" in my own posture and changes in my flexibility, I have come to realize the importance of stretching as part of my own personal daily routine.

I have designed the Morning Cup combination of stretches to be quick and easy. The routine can be done while waiting for the morning coffee to perk or the tea kettle to boil.

I hope you'll also take this routine, or parts of it, with you wherever you go. You can do many of these stretches at work, on the road, or even in your car to help ease, and even prevent, soreness, stiffness, and potential injury. In the second part of the book, you'll get further ideas for adjusting your habits and workspace to give your muscles a happier, healthier, longer life.

All of the stretches here are done in a sitting or standing position, so you won't need a floor mat or any special equipment except a wall and a chair. There's only one exception: The calf stretch is more effective if you use a towel or a belt to pull your foot back.

As with any new exercise program, you should get clearance from your physician or healthcare provider before beginning.

Getting Started

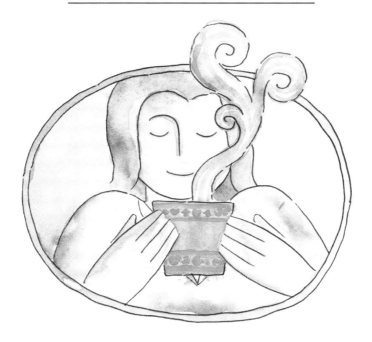

Adding stretches to your daily routine will definitely help you improve your posture and feel better. But don't defeat yourself by thinking you have to suddenly make a radical "lifestyle change." Instead, think of it as a contract with yourself to feel better. You can initiate your new contract by setting up a simple stretching schedule and sticking to it.

In therapy, when we are educating a patient on her injury, we can identify the muscles that are stiff and sore. But we cannot make the stiffness go away until she agrees to study her routine and make changes with us. This involves considering the way things are done at home, in the office, and in the car, to find the cause of the problem. We call this "posture and body mechanics."

It's All About Posture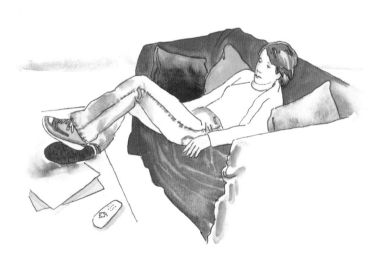

Good posture is the key to alleviating stiffness and aches and pains, regardless of whether you're sitting or standing, at home, or at work. This section will make you more aware of your posture, and will show you how to make necessary changes in the way you do things to prevent those aches and pains from happening in the first place.

Let's do a test called a "slump test." First, sit in a chair. Now slump. I mean really slump. Sit that way for about a minute. Do you feel an ache in the back of your neck, low back, or anywhere else? Now, sit up tall and hold your shoulders back. Which posture feels better? The sitting-up-tall one does. That is because all the bones in your spinal column, instead of all your muscles and ligaments, are supporting your upper-body weight. (If sitting up straight causes you more pain than slumping, then you are already developing tight muscles that can become "contractures," or permanently shortened muscles, and you need a stretching routine even more!)

✳ *Sitting posture.* People who have to sit for long periods at work or elsewhere often suffer from low-back and neck pain from a slumped posture. If you sit like the person in the picture at left, you could be in danger of having low back problems for years to come.

To improve your sitting posture, sit with your buttocks against the back of the chair or sofa. Add a lumbar roll, which you can make by rolling up a hand towel and placing it behind your back to help maintain its natural curve. Place your feet squarely on the floor.

✳ *Standing posture.* People who have to stand for long periods know that it can be quite tiring. Think about the last time you stood in a long line at the grocery store. If your legs got fatigued pretty quickly, it probably was due to the way you were standing. For correct standing posture, do the posture makeover on page 42, and remember the following tips: Knees should be slightly bent, abdominal muscles tight, shoulders back, and ears aligned over shoulders.

✳ *Sleeping posture.* If you wake up feeling not refreshed, but rather like someone has just beaten you up, you may have a bad mattress or poor sleep posture, or both.

Let's talk about your sleep position. If you sleep on your stomach, you are guaranteed to have neck problems down the road. This is due to the fact that in order to breathe, you have to rotate your head in one direction or the other, and your head winds up in this rotated position for long periods. A more correct posture is to sleep either on your side or back. In side sleeping, you can place a pillow between your knees, which keeps the spine in a neutral position. Or you can hug a pillow in front of you, which keeps the shoulders from rotating too far to the front, thereby twisting the low back. When sleeping on your back, you should place a pillow under your knees to alleviate low back pain. (If you have knee pain, this is not advised.)

Some Practical Tips

 Pick one day to start, then do it. The hardest part of starting any new program is just that—starting. So commit to begin on a certain day, and stick to it. Make the decision that this is for you, to help you feel better, that you deserve 15 minutes for yourself.

After you've committed to begin, decide how often and when you will perform the stretches. To get the most benefit, you should do the routine every day. Morning is a great time to stretch. Evenings are good, too, to help relax and wind down after the work day. Once you begin to see results—a little more flexibility, less pain and stiffness—you will look forward to doing the stretches, which will make working them into your day even easier.

The good thing about this routine is that while it is designed to balance all major muscle groups, you can pick out specific stretches and do them just about anywhere, any time. Say that you are at your desk and your shoulders and neck start to ache—do a few neck stretches. It will not hurt you to stretch several times a day.

Rediscover your breathing. Breathing is an important part of stretching. Breathing provides oxygen. Oxygen is carried by the blood to the muscles to help get rid of the toxins that make you stiff and sore. Tight muscles are just that—tight. You stretch to help lengthen the tight muscles. If you hold your breath while you stretch, you cannot get the oxygen and the blood to the muscles to help get rid of those toxins. So, breathing and stretching go hand in hand. We've all been told when we're stressed to "stop and take a deep breath." There really is scientific evidence that the deep breath helps reduce muscle tension. I'll tell you more about breathing in the next section.

 Pay attention to position. When stretching, you want to make sure that you are stretching in the right way. A popular method advocated for years was bouncing during stretching. However, over time,

Balancing the Body

Think of the body as a rubber band. Sagging on one side of the band creates tension on the other side. (Think of a pregnant woman). As we get older and our posture starts to deteriorate, aches and pains begin to develop in the neck and back region. Stretching the chest and the hips on the opposite side of the body can help ease that pain.

I designed the routine in this book as a complete series of stretches to help you get your body in balance. Learning and maintaining proper posture and body alignment are the first steps toward achieving "body balance," and it is where stretching can have the most impact.

we have discovered that bouncing does not cause the muscles to relax; in fact, it actually makes them tenser.

Now we teach a slow, long stretch to help lengthen the muscle. Since you're holding the stretches longer, you want to make sure that you are in the right position so as not to injure any joints. If you are not able to get into any of the positions, do your best to get as close as possible, but don't strain. Remember we are not all built the same. Also, be sure to notice the "Extra Attention" sections offered with some of the positions, which tell how to modify the stretch to make it easier, or in some cases, more challenging.

 Listen to the pain. Pain should never be ignored. It can be a warning sign that something is seriously wrong. A dull ache usually comes from the muscles and is often associated with tension from stress.

You should not feel pain when you do these stretches. The adage, "No pain, no gain" was tossed out several years ago. You should feel the stretches, but not feel pain. If you do have pain, you are stretching too far and should back off until you feel at most a mild discomfort. As you stretch, the discomfort may turn into a burning or tingling. That is okay as long as it is not painful. The discomfort should feel good, like you have hit on the spot that is tender. Remember the stretches that give you this feeling; they are the ones you will want to carry with you to work or on the road, to help work on those chronic sore spots.

Hold that stretch! Not even healthcare professionals agree on how long to hold stretches. The prevailing opinion is to hold each stretch for 30 seconds, and do one or two stretches in each position.

I have carefully selected stretches that address all muscle groups in one 15-minute program. If you have time, you can perform each stretch more than once, holding it for up to one minute. Follow the entire routine with a relaxation exercise (see page 56), and when you're done, you will feel like you've been to the spa.

Take it slow. The Morning Cup stretching program is designed for everyone. Beginners should start the program slowly. Remember, it was the tortoise who won the race, not the hare. The best piece of advice that I can offer beginners is this: You will be more successful starting slowly and gradually, then adding intensity, than if you try to do too much, too soon, and wind up too sore to continue.

Don't get discouraged if you do not do the routine every day. Exercise is something that we pick up from time to time, or when we start to feel bad again. However, you will be surprised when you see how much better you feel if you can do the stretches daily. Your posture—and your whole attitude—will change.

If you are a woman with osteoporosis, the stretches will help you maintain your posture and minimize the effects of the disease. If you have arthritis, the routine can help decrease morning stiffness and increase your flexibility.

If you are interested in improving your workspace and work posture, this book has lots of tips and suggestions.

If you are an athlete, the routine offers a safe guideline for stretching all of your muscles.

If you find that one part of the routine is too hard, then just do what you can. If it is too easy, then challenge yourself with the alternative stretches in some of the "Extra Attention" boxes throughout the book.

Once you have familiarized yourself with the routine, you can use the "Routine at a Glance" on page 79 and the audio CD at the back of the book to simply prompt yourself as you go along. Just keep in mind that the main goal is to stretch and have fun doing it.

Breathing

What kind of breather are you? Breathing is basic to stretching because it provides your body with the oxygen your muscles need to help get rid of the toxins that make you stiff and sore. Good deep breathing comes from the diaphragm (belly area), but many people, women especially, breathe too shallowly, using primarily the chest muscles.

Maybe we women have gotten so used to holding in our stomachs that we've forgotten how to breathe with our bellies. It is important to be aware of the way you breathe, so you can make sure you are inflating all of the air spaces in your lungs. Breathing this way allows you to take a good deep breath, as opposed to a shallow breath using your chest muscles.

To see which type of breather you are, place one hand on your chest and one on your belly, and just breathe naturally. Which hand moves the most? If you answered that "neither one moves much," or that "the chest hand moves more," you are a chest breather: You use your chest and upper neck muscles to breathe. If you answered "belly," then you are using your diaphragm to breathe and are expanding your lungs fully.

The right way to breathe. In a comfortable sitting position, place your hands on your lower ribs. Take a slow, deep breath in through your nose and try to make that breath push out your hands, while at the same time keeping your shoulders relaxed. Then breathe out slowly through your mouth. Your hands should move in with the rib cage. If you are experiencing the reverse effect on your hands, the next time you breathe out, try gently pushing the air out with your hands. Repeat until deeper "belly breathing" feels more natural to you.

Once you practice breathing this way, you will be able to use this technique while you perform the stretches. Remember, it is important to breathe during the stretches to supply yourself with the oxygen your muscles need to stay clean, healthy, and flexible!

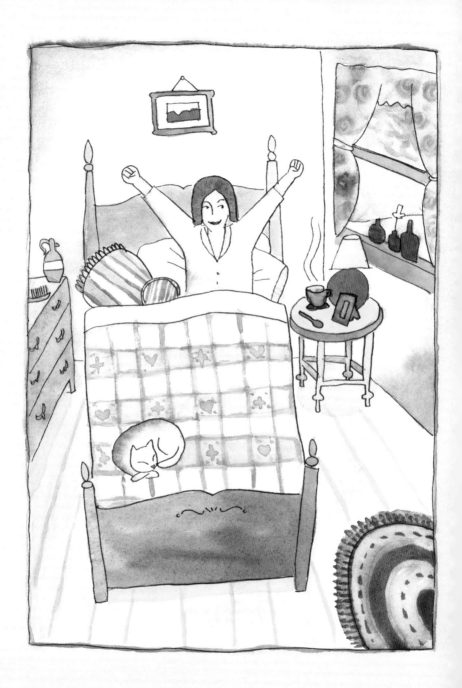

The Routine

Simple stretches to make you feel better every day

What follows are simple stretches that can be performed in 15 minutes. The audio CD in the back of this book will lead you through the routine in exactly that amount of time. But please read the book carefully and study the pictures of the stretches before trying the CD. Remember that proper position is vital to protecting your posture. Remember too, that to effect beneficial change in your muscles, you should hold your stretches for 30 seconds unless instructed otherwise.

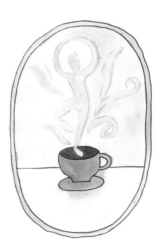

Warm-up

Here's a warm-up breathing sequence that will help prepare your body for stretching.

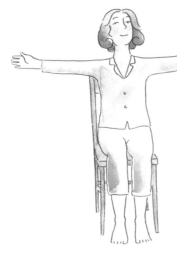

1. Sit with your feet on the floor.
2. Take a slow, deep breath in toward your belly and lift your arms to the ceiling.

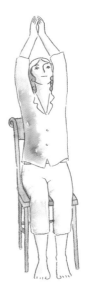

3. Hold the position for one second.
4. Exhale slowly while bringing your arms back down.
5. Repeat three times.

Do You Drink Enough Water?

You can sweat up to four pounds of fluid per hour while exercising in warm weather. That's about 16 paper cups worth of water! If you don't drink enough fluids while exercising, you will experience early fatigue, higher body temperature, loss of muscle coordination, and decreasing ability to concentrate on your workout or game. Even slight dehydration can lead to a less effective exercise session and poor performance.

The fact is, most people are dehydrated. Our bodies need generous amounts of water to stay healthy because we are made mostly of water. For optimal athletic performance and quick recovery, it's important to drink water before, during, and after exercise.

To perform at your best, always begin your athletic event or exercise session well-hydrated. You want the water in your muscles' cells, not in your stomach and bladder, when you begin. Drink at least 16 ounces (two cups) of water one to two hours before beginning exercise, and then weigh yourself. During exercise try to drink five to ten ounces of water every 15 to 20 minutes or more. After exercise, weigh yourself again and drink 16 ounces for every pound you lost during your workout. Another way to see if you are hydrated is to check the color of your urine. If it's the color of lemonade, you're okay, but if it's the color of apple juice, you need water.

Nose-to-Armpit Stretch

This stretch focuses on muscles from the back of the neck to the shoulder blade.

1. To begin, sit in a comfortable chair with your feet on the ground.

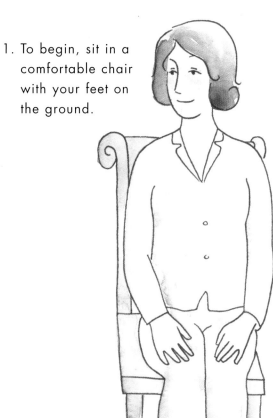

2. Let your arms drop to your sides, hands on lap.

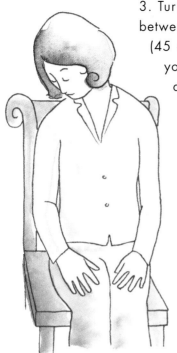

3. Turn your head halfway between the front and the side (45 degrees), and slowly drop your nose down to your armpit.

4. Hold for 30 seconds.

5. As you breathe out, advance the stretch a little further.

6. Return your head to the front, and repeat to the other side.

You should feel the stretch on the side opposite the one you are turned to. For instance, if you are turned to the right, you are stretching the left side.

Extra Attention

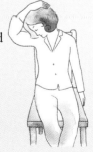

To make this stretch more challenging, gently place one hand (on the same side your face is turned toward) on the top of your head, and anchor the hand from the side you are stretching to the chair. Then perform the stretch.

Take this stretch to work with you.

How Long Should You Hold a Stretch?

Disagreements in this area are common, and really have to do with your choice of stretching environment. Typically, in exercise classes where the stretching is used as a warm-up for a different type of exercise, the stretching is held for a short period of time (10–15 seconds). For instance, the recommended stretching guidelines the American Council on Exercise advise is 10–30 seconds. However, physical therapists and physicians often advocate stretching for a longer period of time, to really make a difference in the length of the muscle tissue. You may have heard the terminology "prolonged static stretching," or "low-load long duration stretching," to refer to these stretching holds. Longer duration stretching guidelines have in fact been adopted by the American College of Sports Medicine and the American Academy of Orthopedic Surgeons. What this all means to you is that, if you are stretching prior to a workout, you may perform the stretches for a shorter length of time. But if you are using the Morning Cup routine by itself, you should hold the stretches for a longer period of time (30 seconds) to really make a change in the length of the muscular tissue.

Ear-to-Shoulder Stretch

This stretch is for the tight neck muscles you get from working at a desk, being in stressful situations, or talking on the phone.

1. Sit in a comfortable, but upright, position.

2. Gently move your ear toward your shoulder until you feel a slight discomfort.

3. Hold this stretch for 30 seconds while continuing to breathe from the diaphragm.

4. As you breathe out, advance the stretch a little further.

5. Return your head to the front, and repeat to the other side.

You should feel the stretch on the opposite side. (If your head is leaning to the left, you should feel the stretch on the right.)

This is a great stretch to do after sitting at your desk for long periods, particularly if you use the phone a lot.

Extra Attention

To make the stretch more challenging, or if you don't feel it, gently place one hand (on the same side your face is turned toward) on the top of your head, and anchor the hand from the side you are stretching to the chair.

Shoulders Round and Grasp

This stretch is for the muscles in the upper back between the shoulder blades, where rounded shoulders can lead to tension build-up.

1. Sit in a comfortable, but upright, position.

2. Lock your hands together, and place them out in front of your shoulders.

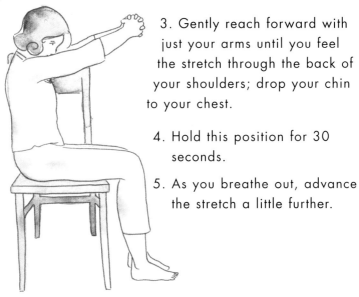

3. Gently reach forward with just your arms until you feel the stretch through the back of your shoulders; drop your chin to your chest.

4. Hold this position for 30 seconds.

5. As you breathe out, advance the stretch a little further.

Extra Attention

This is a great stretch to do at your desk after you have been sitting for awhile.

Cat and Camel

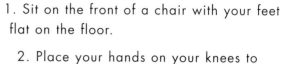

This stretch is a great tension reliever, especially after sitting at a desk or in a car for a long time.

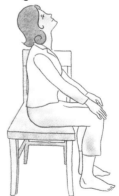

1. Sit on the front of a chair with your feet flat on the floor.

2. Place your hands on your knees to support your lower back.

3. Beginning with your neck, slowly let your head drop toward your chest, then round your shoulders and arch your upper back, lifting your shoulders to the ceiling.

4. Hold this for 30 seconds.

5. As you breathe out, advance the stretch a little further.

6. Slowly exhale and lift your head up; pull your shoulders back followed by a slight arch in your low back. Hold this position for 30 seconds.

Extra Attention

Make sure when you do this stretch that you do not move too far in each direction. It is supposed to be a very gentle stretch to help align the entire back. Always end with the upright position, and try to keep this position as you go through your day.
Take this stretch to work with you.

Knee-to-Chest Stretch

This stretch is great for those aching low back and buttocks areas.

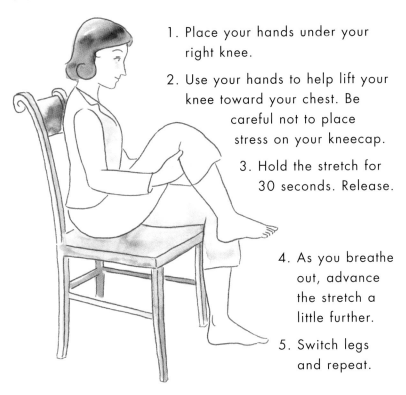

1. Place your hands under your right knee.

2. Use your hands to help lift your knee toward your chest. Be careful not to place stress on your kneecap.

3. Hold the stretch for 30 seconds. Release.

4. As you breathe out, advance the stretch a little further.

5. Switch legs and repeat.

Extra Attention

If this stretch is difficult in the sitting position, you can also do it first thing in the morning, lying on your back. Don't feel this stretch? Arch your low back and pull your shoulders back as you do the stretch. This will help lengthen the muscle.

Knee to Opposite Shoulder

This one is great for a muscle in the middle of the buttocks called the piriformis. It can become tight and cause a lot of pain down one leg.

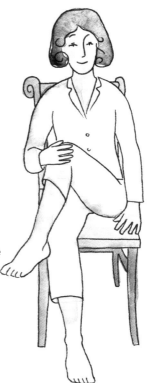

1. To begin, sit on the front edge of the chair.

2. Using your hands, grab your knee and slowly pull it toward your chest and over to the opposite shoulder.

3. Hold this stretch for 30 seconds.

4. As you breathe out, advance the stretch a little further.

5. Repeat with the other leg.

Extra Attention

If you find this stretch difficult to do in the sitting position, you can also perform it lying on your back. Don't feel it? Arch your low back and pull your shoulders back.

Wrist Extensors

This is a stretch for the back of the forearms and wrists. It will feel especially good if you sit at a desk and do a lot of typing. Do this very gently if you have arthritis of the wrists or hands.

1. Sit on the edge of your chair.

2. Begin by straightening out your right arm in front of you.

3. Gently drop your hand toward the ground as if someone is going to kiss the back of your hand. With your other hand, gently hold the dropped hand in position. You should feel this stretch through the top of the forearm.

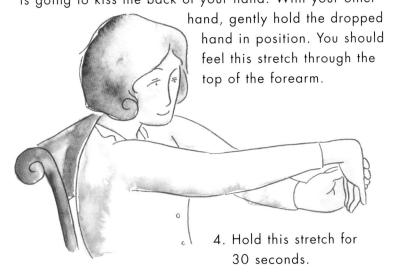

4. Hold this stretch for 30 seconds.

5. As you breathe out, advance the stretch a little further.

6. Repeat with the other arm.

Wrist Flexors

This is a stretch for the palm side of the forearms and wrists.

1. Sit on the edge of your chair.

2. Begin by straightening your arm in front of you.

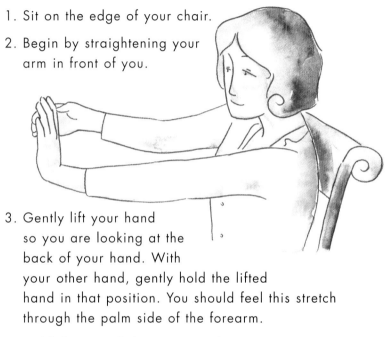

3. Gently lift your hand so you are looking at the back of your hand. With your other hand, gently hold the lifted hand in that position. You should feel this stretch through the palm side of the forearm.

4. Hold this stretch for 30 seconds.

5. As you breathe out, advance the stretch a little further.

6. Repeat with the other arm.

Extra Attention

If these stretches feel good, but they are not strong enough, you can gently pull on the hand with your other hand. Be careful, though, to pull through the palm area only, not the fingers.

Bear Claw

This stretch is for the inner muscles of the palm of the hand. This is also an exercise that we use to help combat carpal tunnel syndrome.

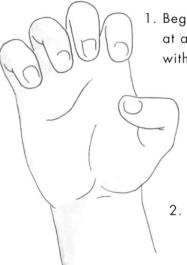

1. Begin by flexing your fingers at all of your knuckles, but without making a fist.

2. Advance the fingers to touch the base of the palm.

Extra Attention

If you have arthritis, remember to move within a pain-free range. Also remember that this range may be different each day. Do not force any position.

3. Open the hand.

4. Touch the tip of the
   index finger with
   your thumb.

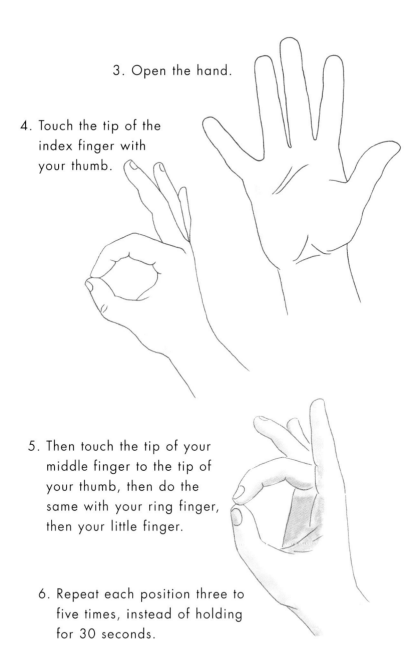

5. Then touch the tip of your
   middle finger to the tip of
   your thumb, then do the
   same with your ring finger,
   then your little finger.

6. Repeat each position three to
   five times, instead of holding
   for 30 seconds.

Hamstring Stretch

This is a stretch for the muscles in the back of the leg. It is also the stretch that people most often perform incorrectly. Follow the steps below carefully, and avoid stressing your back. Don't push past your limit.

1. Sit on the edge of the chair.

2. Place one leg up on another chair.
   Make sure that your knee is flat.

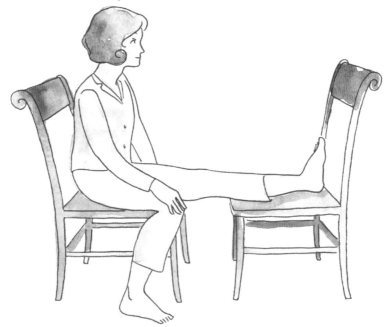

3. Gently arch your low back, sitting up straight and tall.
   Do not lose this position.

4. Gently lean forward until you feel the stretch from your knee to your buttocks. If you do not, then gently lean forward until you feel the stretch, keeping that arched back and tall shoulders.

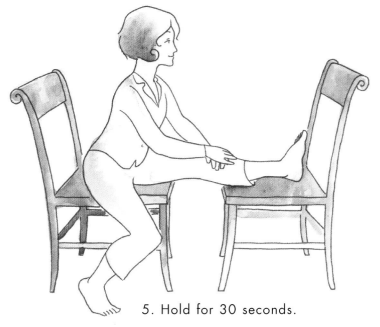

5. Hold for 30 seconds.

6. As you breathe out, advance the stretch a little further.

7. Return to the upright position; repeat with other leg.

Extra Attention

Be careful not to bounce with this exercise. If your shoulders start to become rounded, return to the beginning position and start over again.

Your back should remain perfectly straight during this stretch, and you do not have to lean very far to feel the stretch in your muscles.

Calf Stretch

This stretch has two parts to be sure you completely stretch your calves. To perform this with maximum benefit, you will need a towel or a belt.

Part One: 1. In the sitting position, place your leg up on a chair with your knee straight.

2. Place the towel or belt around the ball of your foot.

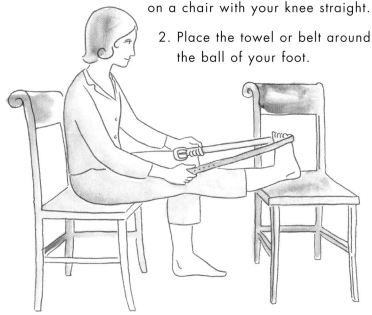

3. Keeping your knee straight, gently pull back on your foot until you feel the stretch in the back of the lower leg.

4. Hold this stretch for 30 seconds.

5. As you breathe out, advance the stretch a little further.

6. Return to the starting position and switch legs.

Part Two:

1. In the sitting position, place your leg up on a chair, but this time with your knee bent.

2. Place the towel/belt around the ball of your foot.

3. Keeping your knee slightly bent, gently pull back on your foot until you feel the stretch in the back of the lower leg.

4. Hold this stretch for 30 seconds.

5. As you breathe out, advance the stretch a little further.

6. Return to the starting position and switch legs.

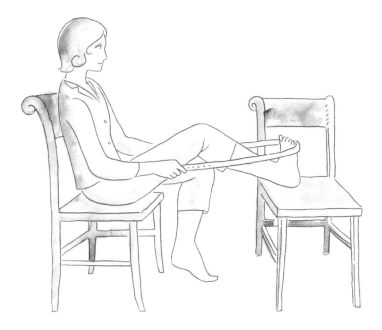

Standing Doorway Stretch

This exercise is good for stretching chest muscles that can get tight from working at a desk, or from poor posture that causes rounded shoulders.

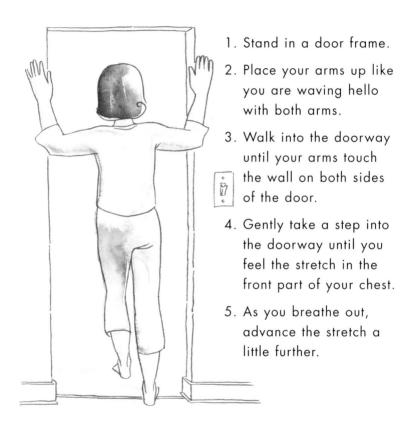

1. Stand in a door frame.

2. Place your arms up like you are waving hello with both arms.

3. Walk into the doorway until your arms touch the wall on both sides of the door.

4. Gently take a step into the doorway until you feel the stretch in the front part of your chest.

5. As you breathe out, advance the stretch a little further.

6. Hold this position for 30 seconds.

7. Repeat.

Side Stretch

This stretch is for the muscles in the abdomen called the obliques. It also stretches tight low back muscles that result from sitting for a long time.

1. Stand with your knees slightly bent.

2. Clasp your hands together and, as you take a deep breath in, lift your arms over your head.

3. As you exhale, slowly bend to the right to stretch the left side of the body.

4. As you breathe out, advance the stretch a little further.

5. Hold for 30 seconds.

6. Repeat by stretching to the left.

Extra Attention

If standing hurts your low back, you can perform this stretch sitting on a firm chair.

Take this stretch to work with you.

Posture Makeover

This is a great stretch, as well as an easy way for you to determine how good your posture is.

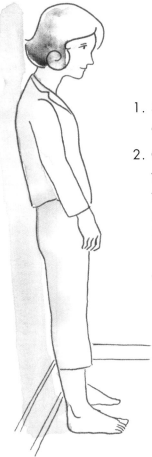

1. Stand with your back up against a wall.

2. Check and see what parts of your body do not touch the wall. If it is your low back, neck, and knees, this is okay. If it is your shoulders and most of your upper back, you could use a posture makeover.

3. To correct your painful posture, gently push your shoulders, mid back, and head back until they touch the wall.

4. Hold this stretch for 30 seconds while taking slow deep breaths.

Now slowly step away from the wall, and try to maintain this posture throughout your day.

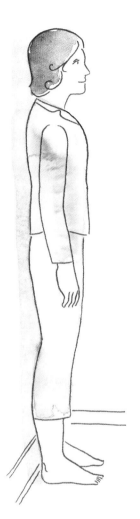

Extra Attention

Do this exercise at least once a day, to see how well you can maintain healthy posture.

Take this stretch to work with you.

Forward Lunge

This stretch is for the front of the hip. If you sit a lot, or have low back pain, this stretch is very important, and often forgotten.

1. To begin, find a chair that you can hold onto.

2. In a standing position, place the chair with the seat near your right knee, and position your left foot near the left back leg of the chair.

3. Place your right knee on the seat of the chair.

4. Hold onto the back of the chair with both hands.

5. Lean forward, bending your left knee slightly, and keeping your right knee on the seat of the chair.

6. Continue to lean forward until you feel a stretch in the front of your right hip and thigh.

7. Hold for 30 seconds.

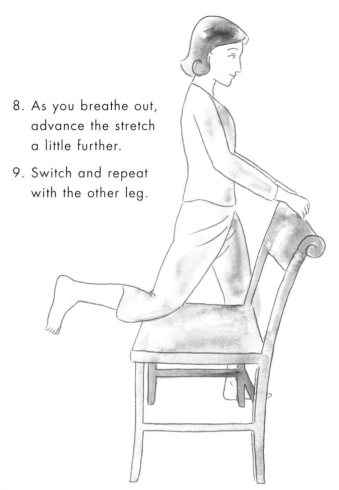

8. As you breathe out, advance the stretch a little further.

9. Switch and repeat with the other leg.

Extra Attention

If you have hip or knee problems (pain in your lower back, hips, or knees) that keep you from performing this stretch, try lying on your stomach and propping up on your elbows, keeping your stomach and hips on the floor or bed.

Quadriceps Stretch

This stretch will work the muscles on the front of the thigh called the quadriceps.

1. Begin by standing and holding onto the back of a chair with your right hand.

2. Gently lift your left ankle toward your buttocks; grab your ankle with your left hand.

3. Gently pull your ankle closer to your buttocks until you feel the stretch in the front of the thigh.

4. Hold this stretch for 30 seconds.

5. As you breathe out, advance the stretch a little further.

6. Switch hands; hold the chair with your right hand.

7. Repeat the stretch with your right leg.

Extra Attention

If you are unable to perform this stretch in the standing position, you can do it lying down. To modify, lie on your stomach and bend one knee, grasping your foot with one hand to increase the stretch. If you cannot reach your foot with your hand, use a towel/belt and place it around your foot to pull the foot gently toward your buttocks.

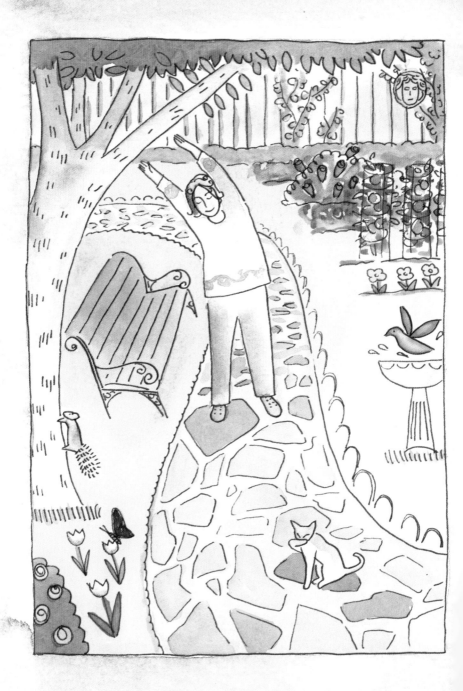

Bringing It All Together

The next sections of this book are designed to help you incorporate the *Morning Cup of Stretching* program into your daily life, and to put it all together with changes in posture and body mechanics to eliminate your aches and pains.

Remember, the routine in this book is simple enough for you to do daily, yet is expandable and adaptable to whatever your own special needs might be. As you learn to bring it all together, you'll find lots of new ways to apply your best combination of stretches, posture, and body mechanics for a healthier, more pain-free life.

Body Mechanics

Remember, posture is something that can change only over time. It has to come from a conscious level and become a habit that is subconscious. To use myself as an example, I can sit and type with the best posture. But then I'll turn around and wash my car and bend incorrectly, placing my back in a poor posture. And when I'm done, I wonder why my back hurts. These changes in posture and stretches work best when we eliminate the things that cause the problems. Just as we have learned bad habits, we can learn good habits, and that is the key to true wellness.

Body mechanics are the positions that we place ourselves in while we are doing daily tasks. The easiest way to remember the key to body mechanics is to remember B-L-T.

B-Bending. Do not bend over to pick up an object! Squat and use your legs, keeping your spine in the upright position. Lifting an object in a bent position can place up to seven times the amount of the weight you are picking up on your spine.

L-Lifting. Do not lift any object that cannot safely be retrieved in the position shown on right. If you cannot pick up the object from a squatting position, the object is too heavy for you to safely pick up, and you should get a second person to help you.

T-Twisting. Do not twist as you are picking up an object, or do not twist while you are carrying the object. This can place a tremendous amount of stress on your low back.

It has been estimated that four out of five adults will experience back pain in their lives. It is the second leading cause of lost workdays for people under the age of forty-five, just slightly behind the common cold. Everyone knows someone who has had back pain at one time or another. Back pain is also the leading diagnosis among chronic pain sufferers. One of the biggest misconceptions about low back pain is that people are usually injured while lifting something improperly. In reality, nearly 85% of all lowback pain stems from unknown causes. This is where proper body mechanics can have a life-changing impact.

Now that you know the staggering statistics, you can make the changes that will help assure your enjoyment of your retirement years. Good body mechanics is the secret. If you make a conscious effort not to bend over even to pick up a sock, you will save thousands of bending repetitions over your lifetime. That will save thousand of pounds of extra pressure placed on your back. That kind of abuse over time can create a "slipped disc," or what is technically known as a herniated disc. However, you do not have to herniate a disc to have pain. Pain from arthritis or from everyday "wear and tear" can be just as debilitating and keep you from getting out of bed.

A Baby Secret

Our poor body mechanics are a product of learned behavior. We live in an instant society, and we are always looking for ways to cut corners. So we end up with injuries.

Think of the baby who has just learned to walk. Watch one some time. Place a baby's favorite toy in front of them on the floor. How do they pick it up? They walk up to the object and almost straddle it. Then they squat, keeping their backs straight, and pick up the object. They do not walk over to the object and bend over and lift it, but actually perform the right movements for body mechanics. Ironically it is as we become stronger that we learn to just bend over and pick up the object.

So let's review one more time.

Good body mechanics require that you keep your body in the correct posture, with your head upright and your shoulders back. Remember: Ears over shoulders, shoulders back and over your hips, knees slightly bent. Good body mechanics require that you keep your back upright while doing daily routines. This requires that you squat to pick up objects, and when the load is too heavy to pick up by squatting, then get help to lift the load.

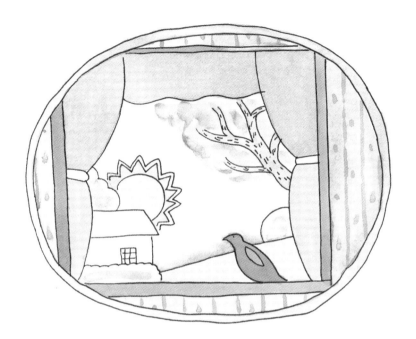

Getting Away from It All

Body mechanics and posture are not the only culprits that cause pain and stiffness. Stress also plays a role in wellness. Stress can make your heart race, your breathing shallow, and your muscles tighten, all of which can cause pain.

So I believe that it goes without saying: To reverse the effects of stress, you need to get away from the stress. Move to a quiet area of the house when you do your stretching routine, or outside to a garden bench. Just get away from the stress, the phone, and anything else that will distract you. Part of the success of this program will revolve around paying attention to your body while you are stretching. And it is difficult to relax when you are still surrounded by the things that are causing the stress or a break in the routine.

This is not to say that you have to break out the incense and burn candles (however, it may help). If the only time you have to stretch is while watching your favorite television show, then stretch during the commercials.

Remember that in the beginning, it may take you longer than 15 minutes to do your stretches. But as you settle into your own routine, you will be able perform all the stretches in that amount of time. And remember that you can do these stretches once a day, twice a day, or as many times a day as you want. You can do the whole routine in the morning and throughout the day, or you can add in the stretches that tackle those tense muscles as they occur.

Explore the *Extra Sip* section to find mini routines that you can do at your desk, in the shower, or at a stoplight to target problem areas. Take time to practice the *Calming Sip* to reduce your stress and tension levels, and to get a peaceful night's rest.

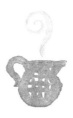

A Calming Sip of Stretching

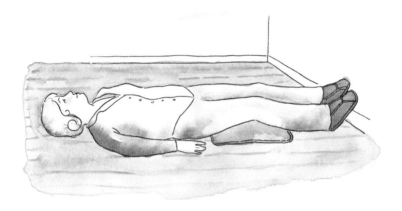

Relaxation is the key to decreasing your muscle tension. But some people find it extremely difficult to relax, especially when they are stressed and need it most. Find whatever it is that allows you to relax, and go out of your way to do it. You may need to be in a completely quiet room; or maybe you find soft music and candles relaxing. Do whatever it takes to find the right elements and environment that work for you. The exercise on the next page is a great one to do after your stretching routine, right before bedtime, or any time you have problems relaxing or falling asleep.

Progressive Relaxation

This is one easy way to practice relaxation. Find a secluded place where you can lie down, or try turning off the lights.

1. Start this exercise by lying on your back. You can place a pillow under your knees for comfort.
2. Take a couple of deep breaths as learned in previous sections.
3. On the third breath, tighten the muscles in your shoulders and neck by shrugging your shoulders; as you breathe out, relax the muscles in your shoulders and neck.
4. Slowly and gently repeat this process three times.
5. On the next breath, tighten the muscles in your arms, forearms, and hands; as you breathe out, let those muscles relax.
6. Slowly and gently repeat this process three times.
7. Now, move to the stomach and low back area. As you breathe in, tighten your stomach and low back muscles; as you breathe out, let those muscles relax.
8. Slowly and gently repeat this process three times.
9. On the next breath in, tighten your buttocks and upper thighs; as you breathe out, relax those muscles.
10. Slowly and gently repeat this process three times.
11. On the next breath in, tighten the muscles in your lower legs and pull back your feet; as you breathe out, relax those muscles and let your feet drop.
12. Slowly and gently repeat this process three times.
13. Now take a couple of deep breaths without tightening any muscles; as you exhale with each breath, you should feel your muscles relax.

A Sip of Stretching at Work

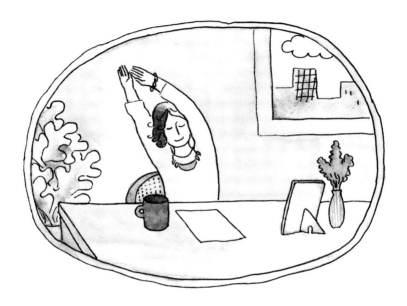

Most of us did not get to design our workspaces, or pick the desks that we have to sit behind for hours on end. In most cases, employers buy one desk and expect it to work for all employees. Obviously, there are problems with this. But there is a way to set up your desk so that it does fit you.

Just as practice and experience help you find the healthy posture that's just right for you, you have to find the posture that fits you at your desk or office. The following tips will help you set up your office space either at work or at home. Most of these ideas can be executed without spending any money.

Organize Your Work Zone

In therapy, we start by assessing what it is a person does at her desk. We ask the question, "What do you do the most?" Type; answer the phone; use an adding machine or calculator; write a lot? Once you identify the tasks that you do most frequently, then you can start to organize your desk according to zones.

The frequent zone. Sit at your desk with your feet comfortably on the ground. Now, place all the objects that you use most frequently in the area closest to you, where you can touch everything without reaching. Some people who answer the phone frequently keep the phone at the back of their desks. This may reduce clutter, but every time the phone rings you have to reach for it. If this happens frequently enough, your repetitious bending and reaching can lead to fatigue and pain in the neck or low back.

The occasional zone. Now place the items that you have to use occasionally throughout your day just past the frequent zone. This may include the stapler, tape dispenser, and similar items.

The family zone. The next zone I like to call the family zone. This is the area that you do not have to reach at all. It's where you should put business cards, family pictures, and other personal, decorative, or infrequently used items.

Once you set up your zones, you'll want to balance them out. If you type and answer the phone a lot, you should place the phone

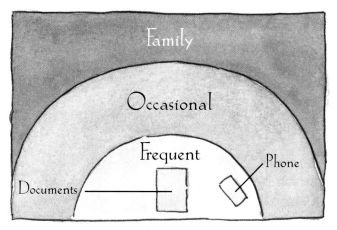

on one side, and a document holder on the opposite side or center. To make this even more effective, get a headset for your phone. Often employers have a couple lying around that are not in use. If you work from home or are on the phone a lot, these can be purchased for most phones for under $15. Using a headset allows you to type and answer the phone at the same time without placing your neck in jeopardy.

Extra Attention

Using a document holder helps keep your neck in the upright position. Document holders in the form of metal or plastic stands can be purchased at office supply stores. My favorite document holder is a large, four-inch, three-ring binder set up like an easel, so the wide spine is facing away from me. This gives you a nice slant-topped holder for the top of your desk, so you don't have to bend over to read things. This can reduce the stress at your neck, and help prevent the "dowager's hump" that some office workers get from leaning over their work.

Work on Your Working Posture

Now that you have set up your work zones and made simple changes to your phone and document holder set-up, let's explore some simple guidelines for proper work posture. I will identify what it means when certain parts of your body hurt, how to make your work area work for you, and which stretches to do to help alleviate stiffness and other problems.

Sit at your desk and see if you can accomplish the following:

- Arms should hang relaxed from your shoulders.
- If you use a keyboard, your elbows, wrists, and the home row (the row with the "J") of keys should roughly line up.

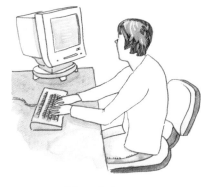

Hurtful

- Your head should be in line with your body, with your chin tucked slightly.
- Your eyes should roughly line up with the center portion of your screen.
- When sitting, your back should be supported by the back of the seat, with the seat height adjusted so that your feet do not hang.
- Your work materials should be within easy reach. Use the frequent and occasional work zone references.

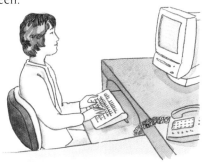

Beneficial

Save Your Back!

Think twice before bending over and picking up that light object. Research has shown that pressures increase tremendously from going from a sitting to a slouched position to a standing bent-over position. Look at the increased disc pressure in the following table to see the increase for that position. Now you can understand why repeated bending over can lead to low back pain, and why adding a lumbar roll can decrease your tension.

Disc Pressure by Activity

ACTIVITY	DISC PRESSURE
Sitting	Increased load by 30%
Walking	Increased load by 15%
Coughing	Increased load by 50%
Jumping	Increased load by 50%
Bending	Increased load by 85%
Lifting 20kg (knees bent)	Increased load by 300%
Lifting 20kg (knees straight)	Increased load by 500%
Sitting with backrest	Decreased load by 10-20%
Abdo muscle contraction	Decreased load by 30-50%

Source: http://www.arthritis.co.za/back.html

Let's talk about what you should correct first. Always start with what you cannot change. If your desk is at a fixed height (as most desks are), you have to adapt your chair first. If you have to raise your chair so that your elbows and wrists are in line with the keyboard while typing, then place something under your feet to get them firmly on the floor. Old phone books taped together are great for steps under your feet. I tape them together so that they do not slide around, or the pages become ripped and worn. Place one phone book under each foot.

If your chair and your desk do not move, see if you can find a chair that can be adjusted. If that's not possible, then place cushions or towels under your bottom to raise you to the appropriate height.

If the chair that you are sitting in is too deep and you have to sit back too far to have your back supported, place a cushion or towel behind your back. Create an inexpensive towel roll to help support your low back while working. Create another towel roll to place in your car. This will keep your back in the right position while you are sitting for long periods of time, keeping the stress off the ligaments and muscles in the low back.

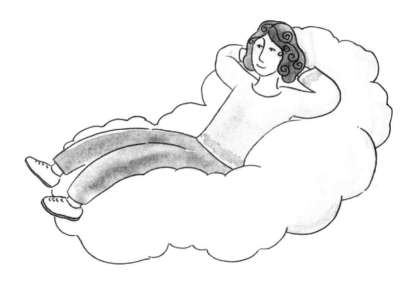

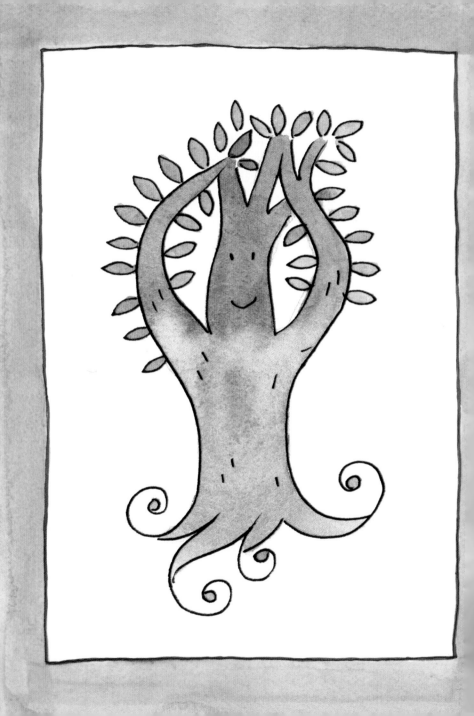

Living a Pain-Free Life

Now that you've learned some of the facts you need to treat your body well, and some of the stretching and posture-correcting tools that will reduce and even prevent aches and pains, let's get a little more specific.

There's no reason why any of us should have to live with pain as long as we have the tools to combat it. In this section we're going to add to your tool kit by looking at some specific areas of your body that may become painful or fatigued at work, or while sitting. If you have any pain in the areas marked on the following pages, use the information in this section to help identify, then eliminate, the causes of the problems. Then throughout the day, use the stretches listed here to help alleviate and prevent pain.

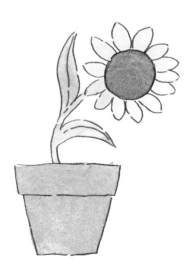

Pain in Areas 1–4:

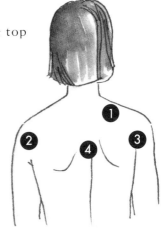

Problem: Pain or stiffness at the top or between the shoulders.

Causes:

- Work surface or keyboard too high
- Backrest too high
- Stress
- Keyboard too close
- Head forward and shoulders rounded
- Arms held too far away from body

Solutions:

- Lower work surface, or raise chair
- Adjust backrest lower to support lower back
- Drop shoulders and hang arms loosely
- Push keyboard drawer away so that arms are in a relaxed position
- Keep head over shoulders, and tuck chin to keep head in correct position

Stretches:

- Posture Makeover
- Nose-to-Armpit
- Ear-to-Shoulder
- Shoulders Round
- Doorway Stretch

Pain in Areas 5–6:

Problems: Soreness at base of the neck or upper back.

Causes:
- Documents are too low
- Screen is too low
- Chair is too low or high

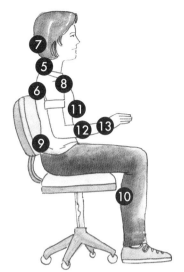

Solutions:
- Raise documents or use a three-ring binder to elevate documents
- Raise screen so that the top of the screen is at eye level
- Adjust chair so that the arms rest naturally and forearms are level with floor

Stretches:
- Ear-to-Shoulder
- Nose-to-Armpit
- Cat and Camel
- Doorway Stretch
- Posture Makeover

Pain in Area 7

Problems: Soreness at top of neck or head held forward.

Causes:
- Visual task too high
- User wears bifocals

Solutions:
- Lower visual task

- Switch to trifocals

Stretches:
- Cat and Camel
- Posture Makeover

Pain in Area 8

Problems: Soreness on the side of neck from head constantly turned either answering phone or looking at document holder.

Causes: Tasks such as answering a phone or typing from a document to one side.

Solutions: Bring work closer to center or alternate placement of work to either side. Use a document holder.

Stretches:
- Ear-to-Shoulder
- Nose-to-Armpit

Pain in Area 9

Problem:
Soreness in the lower back from poor back support.

Causes:
- Backrest too high or low
- Backrest not used
- Forward slumped posture
- Chair too high

Solutions:
- Adjust backrest to firmly support the small of back
- Add a towel roll behind the low back if inadequate low back support
- Sit with proper posture

- Lower chair until forearms are level with floor

Stretches:
- Knee-to-Chest
- Knee to Opposite Shoulder
- Forward Lunge
- Side Stretch

Pain in Area 10

Problem: Lower leg soreness or circulation cut off. This is a serious problem and could lead to blood clots.

Causes:
- Feet not supported on the floor
- Seat pan too deep
- Front of cushion not rounded
- Chair too high

Solutions:
- Lower chair or work surface, or use footrest or phone books under feet
- Place a cushion behind your back so that the front of the chair does not place pressure on the back of your legs
- Change chair to one with a rounded front

Stretches:
- Hamstring Stretch
- Calf Stretches

Pain in Area 11

Problem: Soreness in the top of forearm.

Causes:
- Wrist on table or keyboard when typing

- Keyboard angle too high
- Wrist held stiff
- Typing for extended periods of times without varying tasks
- Elbows stuck out

Solutions:
- Lower keyboard until forearms are level with floor
- Wrists should be in neutral position and not bent in either direction
- Wrists and arms should be in a relaxed position
- Vary tasks to break up long periods of typing
- Allow arms to hang loosely from shoulders (you may have to eliminate any armrests on the chair)

Stretches:
- Wrist and hand stretches
- Doorway Stretch

Pain in Areas 12–13

Problem: Soreness at the outer area of the forearms.

Causes:
- Elbows stuck out
- Keyboard at wrong angle
- Wrist is bent to reach function or cursor keys
- Over-stretching to reach function keys
- Striking keys too hard

Solutions:
- Turn keyboard to straighten wrists
- Move the arms so that the wrist does not have to bend
- Relax work style

Stretches:
- Wrist and hand stretches
- Doorway stretch

Around the House

Proper body mechanics can be a real chore during household activities. Frequently I have to demonstrate body mechanics for people that have pain and stiffness to keep them from continually injuring themselves. The most common areas that cause pain during household activities are: Unloading the trunk of a car, dishwasher, or dryer; and vacuuming. These are the activities that cause the most pain for most people with back pain. Here are some helpful hints.

When unloading the trunk of a car, first bend your knees and tighten your stomach muscles, then pull the object close to you before lifting it. To unload the dryer, squat and move all the clothes to a basket, then transfer that basket to a height where you can fold the clothes either standing or sitting. To unload the dishwasher, squat and move all the dishes to the counter. Stack like items such as plates and then lift. Place them in the cupboard as a unit. This will save on the number of times you are lifting objects.

Vacuuming is one of the most difficult household chores. Just think what your vacuum is doing. It is sucking on your floor. Now examine how most people vacuum, by standing in one position and moving the vacuum in random patterns. Is it any wonder you feel it in your back?

The best way to vacuum is to tighten your stomach muscles and start walking. Walk the length of the area you are vacuuming and then reverse and walk backwards. This will feel better, and give you aerobic benefits too.

An Extra Sip

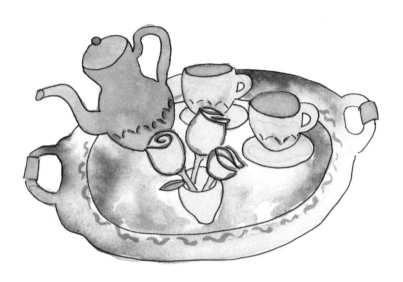

I know that I have covered a lot of ground, and some of it may be confusing. So the best advice is to keep it simple. To summarize:

 The routine. You can use this routine as a stand-alone program, or you can use this stretching routine before any other forms of exercise. You can perform the entire routine before going to work, and then perform the specific routines for those aches and pains that develop at work.

Your posture. Keep your posture simple. Do the posture makeover every day and keep track of your progress. You will see that when you initially start out, your shoulders and low back are really far away from the wall. After several days, you will see that when you back up to the wall, you will just need minor adjustments.

 Your body mechanics. Remember the B-L-T when doing your basic body movements. Do not bend at the waist to pick something up. Do not lift any object in the bent position. And do not twist with the object after you have lifted it.

 Relaxation. Practice relaxation. You will be surprised to see how much tension you are holding in your muscles without knowing it. Until you practice how to relax them, you may not even know they are tense or contracted.

 Organize your workspace. Use inexpensive items such as phone books for footrests, three-ring binders for document holder easels, and towel rolls for lumbar supports to get you in the proper position. Use the frequent, occasional, and family zones to set up your desk to minimize how often you have to reach for things.

 And finally, stretch. You will feel better afterward. I guarantee it. As you're stretching, allow your mind to become quiet and clear, and explore the tightness of your muscles. As those tight muscles relax, you, too, will relax. It's a great feeling.

Mini Routines to Go

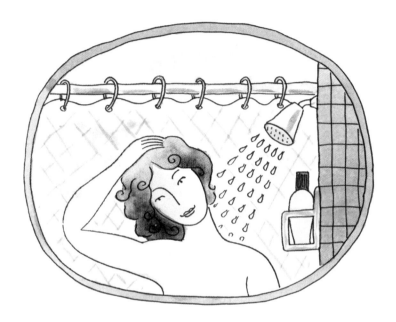

Use these mini routines to target the areas that need the most attention. Remember, these routines can be done in the bathtub, shower, during a pit stop on a long road trip, or at work. If you have pain in a specified area, try all the stretches listed. It may turn out that only one or two really give you that tingling "got it!" feeling that comes when you work a kink out of an especially tight spot. Let your body tell you in this way which are the best of the recommended stretches to take with you and repeat, whenever you feel muscle tension, wherever you are.

Pain in the neck area:

- Ear-to-Shoulder
- Nose-to-Armpit
- Shoulders Round and Grasp
- Cat and Camel
- Standing Side Stretch
- Standing Doorway Stretch

Pain in the low back area:

- Cat and Camel
- Knee-to-Chest
- Knee to Opposite Shoulder
- Hamstrings
- Calf (Parts 1 and 2)
- Forward Lunge
- Quadriceps Stretch
- Standing Side Stretch
- Standing Doorway Stretch

Pain in the forearms:

- Wrist Extensors and Flexors
- Bear Claw
- Standing Doorway Stretch
- Cat and Camel

Travel Tips

We all experience tightened muscles when we stay in one position for a long period of time. People who travel a lot often ask me what to do to avoid the stiffness that can accompany the trip. Here are some general tips to combat stiffness.

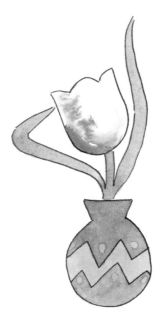

If you're in a car:
- Stop every hour or so, get out of the car and stretch. Work your arms, ankles, and torso, and take a short walk.
- If you can't stop, stretch in your seat. Tighten your calf muscles, hold for three counts, and release. Do the same for your thigh muscles. Roll your shoulders backward and forward a few times. Keep a loose grip on the steering wheel. Clenching it too tightly will tire your hands, wrists, and arms.

If you're in a plane:

Every now and then, get out of your seat and walk down the aisle.

While sitting, tense and release the muscles in your legs and buttocks. Roll your shoulders backward and forward, and wiggle your fingers and toes.

When you put your luggage in the overhead bin, stand out in the aisle so you don't have to twist your back to get the bag over your head and into the compartment.

About the Author

A native of Reno, Nevada, Beth Pierpoint has spent her 20-year career in health and fitness. The past 10 years of her work as a physical therapist have been focused on helping people learn to live free of pain, with maximum functional ability. As an instructor, she has educated people nationwide about healthy lifestyles through fitness activities on land and water. She has worked with many charitable organizations including the Arthritis Foundation and National Multiple Sclerosis Foundation, to help further the cause of fit living for Americans with disabilities. She received an Outstanding Research Award by her physical therapy peers for research in aquatics and has been involved in the development of new robotic technology that will revolutionize recovery for patients suffering from diseases such as stroke, multiple sclerosis, and spinal cord injury. She is currently a member of the Alabama Physical Therapy Association and the American Physical Therapy Association; she also serves on the Alabama Department of Public Health's Task Force for Arthritis Education.

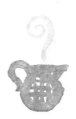

The Routine at-a-Glance

Warm-up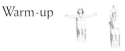

Nose-to-Armpit Stretch

Ear-to-Shoulder Stretch

Shoulders Round and Grasp

Cat and Camel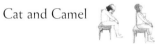

Knee-to-Chest Stretch

Knee to Opposite Shoulder

Wrist Extensors

Wrist Flexors

Bear Claw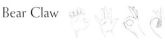

Hamstring Stretch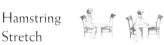

Calf Stretch Part 1

Calf Stretch Part 2

Standing Doorway Stretch

Side Stretch

Posture Makeover

Forward Lunge

Quadriceps Stretch

Tear this page out and post it on your refrigerator or another handy spot for quick reference to your stretching routine.